It Starts With Food

Simple Changes, Incredible Results

By Cathy Wilson
Copyright © 2014

Income Disclaimer

This book contains business strategies, marketing methods and other business advice that, regardless of my own results and experience, may not produce the same results (or any results) for you. I make absolutely no guarantee, expressed or implied, that by following the advice below you will make any money or improve current profits, as there are several factors and variables that come into play regarding any given business.

Primarily, results will depend on the nature of the product or business model, the conditions of the marketplace, the experience of the individual, and situations and elements that are beyond your control.

As with any business endeavor, you assume all risk related to investment and money based on your own discretion and at your own potential expense.

Liability Disclaimer

By reading this book, you assume all risks associated with using the advice given below, with a full understanding that you, solely, are responsible for anything that may occur as a result of putting this information into action in any way, and regardless of your interpretation of the advice.

You further agree that our company cannot be held responsible in any way for the success or failure of your business as a result of the information presented in this book. It is your responsibility to conduct your own due diligence regarding the safe and successful operation of

your business if you intend to apply any of our information in any way to your business operations.

Terms of Use

You are given a non-transferable, "personal use" license
to this book. You cannot distribute it or share it with other
individuals.

Also, there are no resale rights or private label rights
granted when purchasing this book. In other words, it's
for your own personal use only.

It Starts With Food

Simple Changes, Incredible Results

By Cathy Wilson

Table of Contents

Introduction

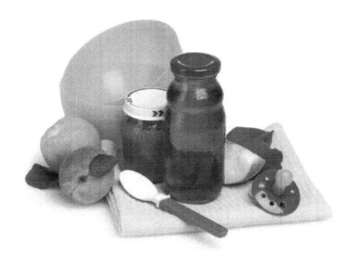

It's all about **CHOICE**. Do you want a nutrition-less simple sugar loaded Twinkie, or a piece of fresh whole grain bread with a dollop of all-natural peanut butter and a crispy crunchy apple?

Both contain the same number of calories but they are so totally different when it comes to the sustainable energy, and essential vitamins and minerals to help your body function optimally and prevent disease.

Perhaps it's not really people that make the world go round, but food?

In this introductory book I'm going to explain how food affects your every day. From energy level and mood, to disease, athletic performance, work production, and overall life satisfaction.

Heck, food also affects your performance in the bedroom! I'm sure you're open to *anything* that'll improve upon satisfying your partner! lol

Like it or not the fuel you fill your engine with determines both directly and indirectly determines how healthy you are in the big picture.

Food even plays a role in how you handle inevitable life stress. As a seasoned nutritionist and fitness professional I'm able to take the intricately complex issues of food, and deliver the key take-action factors that give you the ammunition required to make better eating choices.

It's not about munching like a rabbit or trying to be perfect in food choice. The goal is to gather and store the information that clicks with you, and use it to reprogram your eating habits just a tad better than yesterday, closer to where you want to be tomorrow.

A process that takes **COMMITMENT, TIME, PERSEVERANCE, KNOWLEDGE, TRUE WANT, and BELIEF.**

I will deliver the knowledge and inspire you to want, believe, and persevere. The rest is up to you.

Bottom Line - You deserve to live a life that's inspiring, fulfilling, healthy, and really long. I'm willing to help you out if you're ready to open your mind to all the great there is for the taking.

Enough rambling, let's get down to business, shall we?

Chapter 1 - Why Food?
...Physiological/Mental...

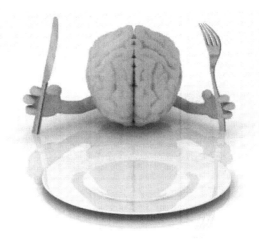

You can't survive without adequate nutrition, nobody can. Your body is mentally and physically dependant on numerous essential vitamins, minerals, proteins, carbohydrates, and fats, to function on a basic level.

Food also affects your social, which we're not going to get into in detail with. But I will mention that making great food choices leaves you feeling and looking fantastic, which affects your overall enjoyment of life, including your social.

When you provide your body with proper amounts of healthy nutrients it performs with a smile.

Your body needs 2-3 servings/day of protein to build lean muscle, provide ample energy, strong nails, healthy skin, and clear thinking, according to *US Nutrition Guidelines*.

To function optimally your body needs to continuously manufacture and control hormones, regulate heart rate, build strong bones and muscle, provide energy, repair muscles after a workout, ensure nutrients get to the right organs via the bloodstream, and ensure harmful wastes and toxins are successfully purged.

Your body runs 24-7 and works the same as your fancy-dance BMW does.

THE BETTER THE FUEL YOU PROVIDE, THE LONGER AND MORE ENJOYABLE THE RIDE!

How does food affect your psychological?

Have you ever wondered how food affects your brain?

According to *Gary Wenk, Ph.D.*, the main interference factor in good health is that your brain rewards you when you fill your belly full of simple sugars, unhealthy fats, and salt. The main ingredients in your list of forbidden foods. Cakes and pastries, fast food hamburgers and fries, convenient and expertly packaged boxed dinners, short-term sugar energy sodas, and sweets and candies we often munch on because we're bored or emotionally taxed, are exactly what your brain wants more of.

All or nothing to is how it works. Foods containing these ingredients have a mental addiction quality directed by your brain. Slowly but surely substantiating and growing your cravings over time, where the more you consume the more you want and honestly believe you need. A cyclic pattern that has no boundaries, according to *Psychology Today* experts.

VIP - Every single calorie you eat directly or indirectly influences your brain.

This connection with food and the function of your brain is easier explained by dividing the foods you eat into 3 categories, according to approximate amounts consumed. Keep in mind the food types and amounts are of course a massive generalization, but accurate enough to serve my purpose.

3 Groups:

*High Dose - Fast Affect
*Slow Affect Over a Period of Time
*Slow to Act - Accumulated Over Time

High Dose - Fast Affect

Foods that Fit: coffee, sugar, nicotine, alcohol, marijuana, magic mushrooms

It depends on how much you take but these foods are immediately reactive and reflect in your physical. Some of these foods have zero affect in low doses. Others can send you through the ringer with just a smidgeon.

Take nutmeg for example. Did you know that nutmeg contains 2 chemicals that your system converts into the street drug Ecstasy? Pretty wild, right? However, in most instances you just get a teeny-tiny bit maybe in your rice pudding or perhaps your holiday beverage. Never enough to give you the full blown response you might get if you doped up on the drug itself.

If you decided to eat a 1 kg tub of nutmeg you'll definitely get a nasty physiological response. Probably sitting on the potty with the runs for about a week and perhaps hallucinating so you truly believe you can fly if you jump off the top of your apartment building.

SERIOUSLY - DON'T DO IT PLEASE!!!

Slow Affect Over a Period of Time

Foods that Fit: various amino acids, high sugar carbs like bagels, potatoes and rice, donuts, eggs, chocolate, cakes, and water soluble vitamins

Some foods take time to affect your brain, usually over a few days or weeks.

Pre-cursor-loading is what many experts call this. What these foods do is trick the set transmitter system, normally to improve its function for your brain.

A prime example without solid scientific backing, is the notion that tryptophan in turkey will make you dopey in large quantities. In order for any food to affect the brain it's got to come across to the right place and in the precise amounts.

The shortcoming with tryptophan is it has difficulties crossing your blood-brain barrier, according to *WebMD* researchers.

It's the flip side that's interesting and more measurable. What happens when you don't get enough of these foods that affect your over longer periods of time?

Researchers have found not getting enough water soluble vitamins or sugar induces chemical changes in the brain after just a few days, which can affect mood, energy, and thinking. Still hard to measure because they take time to cause noticeable changes to your brain.

Slow to Act - Accumulated Over Time

Foods that Fit: antioxidant rich foods like berries, brightly coloured fruits and veggies, fish, olive oils, aspirin, spices, caffeine, chocolate, nicotine, steroids, nuts, liquor, and legumes

These slow out of the starting gates, lifetime dosing food nutrients take time to affect your brain, and accumulate over time in your system.

The affects aren't immediate like an energy spike or fast mood change. These benefits are seen over time, slow and progressively. Think of it like you might an after-the-fact scenario.

Experts believe these foods act as protectors over time against oxygen, which gets deadlier as the clock ticks.

FACT - By taking in oxygen we age, and of course by aging we eventually die.

TRUTH BACKED BY PSYCHOLOGY TODAY - Research studies show people who eat more foods rich in protective antioxidants and eat less food in general, tend to live longer.

Technically if you want to slow the aging of your brain, you've got to munch on specific foods that trigger particular chemical processes. Of course that's the last thing we think about when looking to get stuffed. We may eat healthy but still go for what tastes and looks good first. You see the destructive and confusing cyclic process here because your brain naturally shouts out to you to eat more sugar, bad fat, and salt. So essentially you've got to battle your brain and overpower it, in order to eat to live longer.

That's **WAY** too much conscious thinking for most people!

How does food affect your physical function?

There's no doubt your life is powered by food. Your food choices affect every single bodily process from breathing, to moving and thinking. Somewhere along the road of evolution humans got sidetracked. We started wanting more, faster, bigger, better, longer, and stronger. We simultaneously rewired our mind and body to accept and even crave unhealthy processed fast foods, sugars, fats, and fattening foods that kill great health.

Deep breath...

Your physical energy levels, muscle strength, endurance, optimal performance level, and speed in which you perform, are all directly affected by the fuel choice for your tank. What you eat and the amount determines how much housework you're going to get done, whether or not you'll hit the gym, if you're going to take the kids to the park, your performance at work, and whether or not your partner's going to get lucky!

It's all about the food.

When you're eating plenty of fresh fruits and veggies, lean meat, and drinking oodles of water, your body runs silky smooth. Less aches and pains appear, injuries are less likely to occur, your attitude will reflect the positive, and you're more motivated to get down with saying active.

On the other hand...

If you are the couch potato candy eater that craves fatty fancy beverages, has fast food as your middle name, and takes pleasure is chowing down a whole tub of triple chocolate ice cream solo, then you're choosing to have a body that runs like you've put diesel fuel in your unleaded tank.

Disease and illness are going to be your every day, energy levels will cease to exist, and you're going to have to muster up effort to drag your butt off your cotton candy couch to use the potty. Not to mention the fact you'll have an increased chance of trading in your granny panties for Depends sooner than most others!

No blaming because it's all about choices, your choices!

Unhealthy food choices like donuts, fried chicken, tempura veggies, chicken wings, fries, Italian bread with butter, and sweet pastries for dessert, are going to set you up on the never-ending roller coaster of spikes and crashes in your health.

By understand all the dangers of crap eating, and flipping your food switch to lean protein, complex carbs, healthy fats, and plenty of protective antioxidants, you're making the brilliant move of choosing to use your fuel to get fan-tabulously healthy, lean and strong.

My Thoughts...

Food really does make your world go round, at least mentally and physically. By acknowledging, learning, and understanding what food does to you directly and indi-rectly in body function and thinking capacity, you'll gain the knowledge required to make better food decisions for you.

It's not about trying to be perfect. That's just a recipe for disaster. What's important is opening your mind to alter-native eating choices that your body physiologically needs, not just what you want.

Over time you're going to see positive change. It won't take long for you to "feel" different and "look" different. Slimmer, trimmer, stronger, and more toned sexy is how you'll look. This helps boost confidence and fuel the fire for more positive change.

Your energy levels will skyrocket and your body will just run better. It's a choice I'll help you make.

Chapter 2 - Key Factors Influencing Nutrition

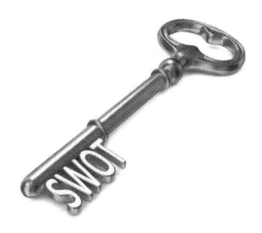

According to the *Cleveland Clinic of Psychology,* understanding why you make specific food choices and what your body needs intrinsically, will help you curb your eating issues, re-programming your mind to eat positively and gain.

Factors that Influence the Foods you shoot Down the Hatch

Food Availability - This factor can be a negative or positive. If your body is physically hungry, rumbling tummy hungry, then having a sub shop nearby is a fantastic thing. You can give your body some healthy nutrition immediately.

On the other hand, when there's food everywhere, this also fuels the fire for overeating, and choosing convenient unhealthy fast foods instead of healthy wholesome ones.

Drive-thru joints are tempting, and it takes a learned self-control to not hit them just because they're in the picture.

Comforting Routines - People need routines in order to function optimally. There's a comfort with routine that sets the mind at ease, relaxes, and makes life more productive. Planning what you're going to eat and when is critical in learning to fuel your body optimally.

Family meals are a great way to do this by supporting family bonding and strengthening social skills. If you've got little ones around you're setting an awesome example providing a healthy meal routinely.

Keep in mind not all routines are positive. For instance, getting into the habit of waking up in the middle of the night to eat munchies every night is NOT a positive routine. Recognizing how to make your routine in eating positive is a quality move.

Physical Health Factors - Many times what you eat is directly reflected in your "in the moment" health. If you're under the weather chances are you're not going to have a ravishing appetite. However, when you're feeling chipper again food intake will creep right back up to your normal zone.

If you happen to notice drastic changes in your natural appetite this may be a signal of a larger issue, one that needs discussing with your healthcare provider.

Cultural Factors - Your ethnic background and upbringing are valid influencers on your daily food regimen. Some cultures are incredibly healthy in eating and others not so much. You need to research yours and learn the positives of your culture, and recognize the eating traits that need changing. Separate yourself from the emotional and look at your specific scenario with an open mind and black and white scientifically proven food facts. A challenge is to re-create your learned cultural food traits and magically transform them better.

There are ways to make a-new recipes from nasty unhealthy, to wholesome and good, without much effort. You've just got to first recognize this, make the decision to adjust things, and take action to make it happen, and repeat!

Social Factors - Your social patterns are likely what gets you into hot water with food. The amount you interact with people socially is directly reflective of what food choices you make, how much you eat, and how often.

Just think about Christmas time when you're managing your schedule to get from one feast to the next to satisfy as many people as possible! You might have brunch at 11 am at your mom's, then scoot to your boyfriend's for lunch at 1, dinner at your dad's around 5, and then off for dessert and drinks at your grandma's for 8.

That's just freaking crazy! But we do it!

The social pressures of throwing your healthy eating habits to the wind and eating WAY more than your physical body needs are overwhelming and dangerous.

Learning to gain control of your social calendar and minimize the situations you know you'll end up overeating in, will only help you learn to get your food cap on straight and keep it on.

Factors of Emotion - Are you someone that rewards yourself with a gynormous chocolate sundae when promoted at work? Or do you reach for your stash of forbidden sweet treats when your hormones take a dive, leaving your feeling alone and worthless?

Do the food choices you make reflect your mood of the day?

Do you use food as an excuse to deal with depression, or going overboard on the Trans-fat loaded deep fried honey garlic chicken wings and beer?

Some people starve themselves because of life emotional triggers. Others turn into a pig-out junk food eating machine. By recognizing your attitude with food on an emotional level, opening your mind to change, and taking action to create new healthy emotional eating habits, you're going to be one step closer to gaining control of your food choices and amounts. Something that will do you very proud.

Food/Nutrition Knowledge - If you don't know the difference between eating a piece of white bread versus brown bread, or that a handful of nuts is more than a serving, it's all but impossible for you to make the healthiest most beneficial food choices for you.

24

It's all about change. Open your mind to learning what's healthy and what's not and giving yourself the opportunity to start making healthier food choices in your every day. There will be a learning curve for sure, one that will have dips and dives, and success and defeat. All you've got to do is commit to gather knowledge forever and you've nothing to lose except pesky fat, and everything to gain.

Economic Reality - There's zero doubt how much green stuff you have in your back pocket influences the foods you shoot down the hatch, a choice with limitation if you're technically poor. A claim supported by *Centers for Disease Control and Prevention.*

Unfortunately in our society many of the healthier food choices, like fresh fruits and meats, and organic, are downright expensive! On the flip side, the Trans-fat load-ed pastries, cakes, boxed dinners, and fast foods, are relatively cheap. So many people are influenced to forgo the healthy eating to fill their belly.

The Canadian Dietician Association states the lower the economic status of a family the increased likelihood for unhealthy eating. Oodles of studies have been conducted to verify this fact.

The Solution - Increased economic stability for our world as a whole, or perhaps better availability for healthy food choices to those families that are less fortunate.

Food Timing - If you skip breakfast chances are you're going to be in a badass grumpy mood, more likely to snack on sugary crap, and my expert guess is you'll likely choose to pig out at lunch because your tank is running on empty. When you are drained willpower simultaneous-ly seems to shoot straight through the window.

25

Your body runs constantly from the moment you wake up till you hit the hay. This means it's constantly burning energy. Eating regular mini-meals throughout the day packed with energizing lean protein, sustaining complex carbs, and oodles of essential vitamins and minerals will give your body and mind the energy it requires for optimal performance.

Choose to keep your tank half full and you're giant steps ahead of the game.

Consequential Factors - Just knowing there are positive and negative consequences in eating sways your food choices. If you are thirsty but trying to get to sleep, it's wise-owl smart to choose a glass of water instead of a coffee or sugar loaded soda, which are stimulants to wake you up not send you to dreamland.

If you're getting set to play hockey and need a snack to boost your energy and decide on a donut, you'll get a short-lived simple sugar induced high, that's going to leave you without energy fast.

A better choice is a piece of whole grain toast with peanut butter and an apple. This provides your system with protein and good carbs for immediate sustained energy, and the ability to re-fuel muscles and build them.

Knowing the consequences of your food choices will help you to forevermore strive to make better ones.

My Thoughts...

These are just a few of the key factors influencing the foods you eat, quantities, and how often. Each life scenario is different. It's important you identify which factors are relevant to your eating habits and create a plan to make positive change where it matters most to you.

As always it's a choice. You can choose to take action and make healthy changes, or ignore everything, hop back up on your worn-out sofa and live the rest of your days eating Ding-Dongs in a sappy state.

Make me smile and choose good health so I can write more books for you!

Chapter 3 - Food Faux Pas

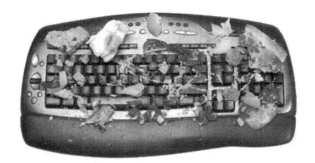

Most people would *like* to make vitamin rich, low calorie, and good fat food choices. Fact is there's a gynormous difference between *wanting* and *doing*. Intentionally or not most of the developed world is making major *faux pas* in eating.

Every poor food choice we make inhibits us from reaching our healthy weight loss and sustainment goals, increases the risk of serious disease, steals precious energy, plays Russian roulette with our volatile blood sugars, triggers depression, enhances mood swings, and steals from our brighter energized future.

THE SOLUTION

I'm going to uncover common eating mistakes that will give you the power to make better food decisions, reaching your health and wellness goals that much sooner.

Eating Issue #1 - Grocery shopping once a week and buying fresh produce.

There's nothing wrong here for the first day or two. However with fresh produce, the fruits and veggies immediately start losing some of their nutrients and protective antioxidants to the oxidation process. Pretty tough to gauge how long the goods have already been collecting dust.

Take Action Pointer - Buy your fresh produce every couple days and don't be afraid to keep frozen on site. Fruits and veggies are flash-frozen. This means at the peak of nutrient rich and ripe freshness they're blasted rock hard. This seals in all the vital nutrients and protects for at least a year.

So don't be afraid to use frozen fruit in your smoothies and snack on frozen peas and corn. All of it will do your body fantastic!

Eating Issue #2 - Fast-Food too many times weekly.

Particularly when juggling work, school, and all the kids team sports, it crazy-butt challenging to time the eating so most of it can happen at home, with a healthy cooler of snacks packed for the road every day.

Just a few years back the National Restaurant Association stats indicated almost 60% of all restaurant activity was take-out, either pickup or delivery. Shocking I know!

A research study conducted at *Harvard University* concluded people getting the majority of their calories from unhealthy fast foods were likely to have a higher BMI than the general populous. In plain English, they were generally fatter.

VIP-Healthy cooking at home makes for happier, healthier, and leaner families.

Take Action Pointers -

*Plan the meals for the week and pick a day to prep as much as you can for healthy eating with the convenience factor.

*Make sure the cupboards are never bare, with oodles of healthy food choices.

*Slow-cookers are a fantabulous way to have healthy tasty meals ready the second you walk through the door.

*Be open to the fact a healthy dinner can be whipped up in 5 minutes, faster and cheaper than the drive-thru. How about scrambled eggs with ham, cheese, and broccoli, with whole grain toast, and fresh fruit for dessert?

Eating Issue #3 - Easy on the packaged crap.

We all know boxed foods, frozen dinners, convenient, and pretty packaged food items aren't the healthiest choices on the block.

When you can keep bread in your cupboard for TWO weeks, what's that telling you? How do you think a muffin lasts a month in the vending machine? They're all loaded with harmful chemical and preservatives, along with synthetic toxic Trans-fat, that's linked to oodles of serious diseases. These fake fats are made in the place of real fat because the shelf life is longer, the appearance of the food is better, and it's ultimately cheaper for the manufacturers. People are knowingly putting their health at risk just to put more money in someone's pocket. This couldn't be more wrong!

Take Action Pointer - Choosing natural healthy whole foods is going to provide your body with the macronutrients for good health. This includes lean protein, complex carbohydrates and healthy fats, along with oodles of essential vitamins and minerals with protective antioxidants. These all help you stay lean, energetic, disease-free, and set to stand the test of time.

Eating healthy grain bread and whole grain rice and pasta, fresh fruits and veggies, fatty fish like salmon and tuna twice a week, and plenty of refreshing water, is a great start to smarter eating.

Eating Issue #4 - Thinking fat loaded plant foods are nasty bad.

Keep moderation in mind because too much of a good thing just isn't. Olives, nuts, and avocados are three high fat plant foods many people steer clear of because they're high-fat and calorie loaded.

According to the *USDA* a 150 gram avocado has about 250 calories, and 22 grams or almost 200 calories of fat! Good news is the fat is healthy unsaturated fat. These plant foods are also high in healthy fiber and protective phytochemicals.

These foods are extremely healthy, just stick to the serving sizes; 1/4 avocado, 3-4 olives, or 1/4 cup nuts.

Take Action Pointer - Make sure you include these health nut foods in moderation. Just be sure to keep the portion size in check and keep the salty nuts away when you're having a beverage or watching the tube. It's just too easy to eat the whole freaking jar without notice.

Eating Issue #4 - Fooling with natural food structure and chemistry.

Are you a potato or apple peeler? Do you drizzle some healthy fat over your veggies and let your garlic "rest" before using? Something we often don't think about is how foods naturally complement one another and then your system.

For instance, eating a little healthy fat, like avocado or olive oil on or with your veggies helps your body absorb healthy phytochemicals.

The fiber and majority of heathy nutrients are hidden in the skin of apples and potatoes. So peeling away is stealing from your food health value.

Eating Issue #5 - Wolfing down dinner like it's your last supper!

I understand life is chaotically fast paced. We always want to do more with less time and naturally this rubs off on your eating style.

Fact: Your stomach and brain are like Dumb and Dumber when it comes to communicating with each other. It can take up to 20 minutes for tummy to signal to your brain the kitchen's closed, and longer still for your brain to acknowledge this and make you feel like you're about to pop.

This makes it **WAY** too easy to make habit of overeating, and realize too little too late, when you're lying on the couch with your pants undone wishing it all away.

Take Action Pointer - Make a point of eating small meals more often instead of the traditional 3 jumbo meals each day. This will help give your body a chance to recognize when you're full or still hungry, and you can adjust.

You can also slow down your chewing and stretch out your meals to at least 20-30 minutes. This'll give Dumb and Dumber a chance to be heard.

Eating Issue #6 - Chickening out on sending your meal back.

Let's say you're dining out for a treat and you got smart and ordered a garden salad with dressing on the side to drizzle, with grilled salmon, and a side of grilled asparagus instead of white bread.

You're heart sinks when the sexpot waiter brings your salad soaked in dressing, the salmon is breaded, and instead of extra veggies you've got white buttered bread.

DON'T use this as an excuse to eat that crap! Your order is wrong, from healthy, to fattening and unhealthy, so send it back.

Take Action Pointer - **IMMEDIATELY** point out to your hunky waiter what you'd like changed in a cutzie manner. He'll obey you and bring your meal fixed.

My Thoughts...

There are so many factors in eating you can adjust for the better. Simple things, even no-brainer moves like tasting your food before dousing it with salt, butter, sour cream, and other fattening condiments are doable steps toward better eating.

*IT ALL STARTS WITH GATHERING KNOWLEDGE!

Sift through this knowledge and pinpoint what marries well with your preferences and tolerances, what's going to inspire you to continue to make positive healthy eating changes, with the purpose of bettering you physically, mentally, socially, and so forth.

Make the time to consider your eating faux pas and **TAKE ACTION!**

Chapter 4 - Main ESSENTIAL Nutrients Your Body Needs and Why?

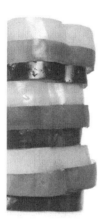

I've no choice but to focus just on the main nutrients your body requires for optimal function. Simply because this is an introductory book and I'd be writing forever and a day if I properly went through each one of them.

This doesn't mean there aren't other important essential vitamins and minerals that you're going to read about here. Just think of this as a solid platform from which to build your **FOREVER** healthy eating platform, your home base.

What's an Essential Nutrient?

According to *The American Journal of Clinical Nutrition*, this is the complete list of essential nutrients:

*Water
*Energy
*Amino Acids - Histidine, Isoleucine, Leucine, Lysine, Methionine, Phenylalanine, Threonine, Tryptophan, and Valine
*Essential Fatty Acids - Linoleic and Linolenic Acids
*Vitamins - Ascorbic Acid, Vitamin A, Vitamin D, Vitamin E, Vitamin K, Thiamine, Riboflavin, Niacin, Vitamin B-6, Pantothenic Acid, Folic Acid, Biotin, and Vitamin B-12
*Minerals - Calcium, Phosphorus, Magnesium, and Iron
*Trace Minerals - Zinc, Copper, Manganese, Iodine, Selenium, Molybdenum, and Chromium
*Electrolytes - Sodium, Potassium, and Chloride
*Ultra-trace Minerals

Essential nutrients are defined as nutrients the body doesn't have the ability to manufacture in adequate amounts. In basic these include essential vitamins, minerals, and protein.

General Consequences of Insufficient Amounts

*PREVENTABLE disease and illness
*Death in extreme cases

What about Carbohydrates?

Interesting to note, the theoretical minimum level of CHO or carbohydrate intake for human adults is zero. Although CHO is the primary fuel source for all living cells, the most cost effective form of body energy, and holds the rights to the main source of plant fiber.

Add to this, without CHO energy readily available in your system for fuel, the body breaks down fat and protein for energy, which triggers ketosis, a dangerous and potentially deadly condition.

As you can see there's expected controversy here. And aside from the technical or scientific reasoning for leaving complex carbohydrates out of the essential nutrient definition, experts still agree base levels are favorable for most people.

We are going to have a look at fat-soluble vitamins, water-soluble vitamins, minerals, protein, and water. I know water is technically classified as an essential nutrient, although it really carries no nutritional value. However, without water for absorption, transportation, and hydration, you're dead meat! I think that's justification for at least summing up the importance of it.

Fat-Soluble Vitamins

Of critical importance is understanding many of these vitamins and minerals are dependent upon one another. For instance, vitamins A, D, E, and K are fat-soluble, stored in tissue for a few days. However if you aren't getting enough vitamin D, or your stores run on fumes, calcium won't get absorbed and bone issues may result.

If you aren't eating enough vitamin K found in sweet potato, carrots, and leafy dark green veggies, your vision may be compromised. The eye will harden and irreversible blindness will be your fate.

You can see the importance of these essential fat-soluble vitamins. Here's a bit of a breakdown for each of them so you can make the best decisions toward eating for better health!

Vitamin A Foods - recommended 5000 IU/day adults

*Carrots (7500 IU/carrot)
*Sweet Potato (20000 IU/med potato)
*Butternut Squash (11000 IU/half cup)
*Kale (20000 IU/cup)
*Leafy Greens (50000 IU/cup)
*Red Peppers (5000 IU/pepper)
*Tuna Fish (700 IU/ounce)

Function

*Boosts Immunity
*Improves Vision
*Gene Health
*Healthy Skin

Consequence Deficiency

*Blindness
*Jaundice
*Tummy Troubles
*Moodiness
*Hair Loss

Vitamin D Foods - recommended 600 IU/day adults - over 10000 toxic

*Milk Products (60 IU/cup)
*Eggs (40 IU/egg)
*Salmon (600 IU/3oz)
*Whole Grain Cereals (90 IU/ounce)

Function

*Assists Calcium Absorption

*Cell Growth and Function
*Optimal Bone Health
*Inflammation Control
*Optimal Immune System Function
*Neuromuscular and Skeletal Function

Consequence Deficiency

*Rickets
*Weak Immune System
*Increased Risk Cancer
*Weakened Bones and Muscles
*Increased Risk Cardiac Arrest/Kidney Stones with Too Much
*Crappy Hair

Vitamin E Foods - recommended 20 mg/day adult

*Spinach (5.5 mg/cup)
*Seeds (10 mg/ounce)
*Tofu (4.5 mg/3oz)
*Avocado (4 mg/avocado)
*Broccoli (2.5mg/cup)

Function

*8 Fat-Soluble Vitamins Deter Oxidation
*Protects Against Cardiovascular Disease, Macular Degeneration, and Various Cancers

Consequence Deficiency

*Increased Risk Disease
*Too Much - Bleeding/Hemorrhaging

Vitamin K Foods - recommended 80 micrograms/day

*Onions/Scallions (30 micrograms/onion)
*Kale (530 micrograms/cup)
*Asparagus (30 micrograms/cup)
*Chilli Powder (3 micrograms/tablespoon)
*Brussels Sprouts (30 micrograms/cup)

Function

*Necessary for Blood Clotting/Protein Health
*May Help Treat Osteoporosis/Alzheimer's
*Could Help Prevent Cardiovascular Disease and Various Cancers

Consequence Deficiency

*Issues Utilizing Protein
*Increased Risk Disease

Note - You don't ever have to worry about overdosing on vitamin K!

Water-Soluble Vitamins

These vitamins scoot out through the body, sometimes too quickly for adequate absorption. This means B-complex vitamins and C vitamin foods need to be eaten regularly.

Cartilage and blood vessel construction is dependent on these vitamins to start, with serious consequences if you fall short, particularly anemia and death.

Vitamin C Foods - recommended 60mg/day adult

*Kale (80mg/cup)
*Strawberries (10mg/berry)
*Oranges (70 mg/orange)

*Tomatoes (25mg/tomato)
*Yellow Pepper (340mg/pepper)

Function

*Manages Blood Vessel, Cartilage, and Scar Tissue Function
*Helps Create Peptide Hormones, Dopamine, Tyrosine, and ATP
*Protective Antioxidant against Disease

Consequence Deficiency

*Anemia
*Easing Bruising and Bleeding
*Slowed Metabolism
*Weight Gain
*Dry Skin
*Swelling Joints
*Weak Tooth Enamel
*Scurvy - Namely Malnourished Adults

Vitamin B-Complex Foods - including Thiamine (B1), Riboflavin (B2), Niacin (B3), Pyridoxine (B6), Folate, Cobalamin (B12), Biotin, Pantothenic Acid

*Cereal, Rice, Pasta, Beans, Legumes, Whole Grain Bread
*Eggs, Red Meat, Clams, Fish, Shellfish, Pork, Poultry, Tuna
*Broccoli, Sweet Potato, Peas, Orange Juice, Spinach
*Cheese, Nuts, Yogurt, Milk Products, Avocado

How Much Do You Need?

Eating a well-balanced diet will provide your system with plenty of Vitamin B-Complex. As you can see you can get it from a diverse range of foods.

Function

*Convert Food into Fuel
*Provide Energy
*Promote Healthy Skin/Hair
*Deters Memory Loss
*Prevents Headache/Migraines

Consequence Deficiency

*Skin Issues - dermatitis, dry skin, bruising, and slow healing
*Extreme fatigue - muscle pain and numbness
*Mental Issues - confusion and moodiness
*Sensitivity to Light
*Anemia
*Tummy Troubles - nausea, vomiting, or diarrhea
*Neurological Issues in Pregnancy - baby can be born with developmental issues

Minerals

Dr. Linus Pauling, Nobel Prize-winner, believes every single health issue you ever face can be traced back to some sort of a mineral deficiency. Pretty powerful words.

It makes sense when you stop to ponder it. When your system doesn't absorb enough iron, you feel tired and cranky. If you aren't getting your quota of calcium, you will eventually end up with osteoporosis.

Never mind what you could-a, should-a, would-a done. Let's focus on the now and what you **ARE** going to do.

COLD HARD FACT - Minerals are something your body and mind requires in adequate amounts for optimal health.

It's sad that almost **NINETY-FIVE** percent of Americans don't munch daily on enough fresh fruits and veggies to get the minerals their body is screaming for. That's according to *Karen Ansel*, registered dietician.

We are going to look at the 5 major minerals you can't be healthy without!

Zinc Foods - recommended

*Pork
*Crab
*Beef
*Oysters

Function

*Fights Infection
*Flu and/or Cold Resistant
*Heal Faster
*Sharpens Senses
*Healthier Pregnancy

Consequence Deficiency

*Weak Immune System
*Dull Taste and Smell
*Wounds Won't Heal
*Growth Issues with Fetus

Calcium Foods - recommended

*Dairy Products
*Calcium Fortified Orange Juice/Other Foods
*Beans
*Spinach
*Broccoli

Function

*Regulates Blood Pressure
*Builds Strong Bones
*Supports Healthy Skin and Hair
*Prevents PMS

Consequence Deficiency

*Weakened Skeletal System - Osteoporosis - Brittle Bones

Magnesium Foods - recommended

*Brown Rice and Pasta
*Bran Cereal
*Swiss Cheese
*Molasses
*Almonds

Function

*Balances Over 300 Internal Chemical Reactions
*Boosts Energy
*Promotes Healthy Cells
*Regulates Blood Pressure
*Supports Strong bones
*Deters Insulin Resistance
*Shuns Away Migraines

Consequence Deficiency

*Abnormal Cell Function
*Increased Risk Disease
*Decreased Energy
*Elevated Blood Pressure

Potassium Foods - recommend

*Baked Potato
*Bananas
*Artichokes
*Raisins
*Tomatoes

Function

*Controls Salt Absorption/Regulates Blood Pressure
*Deters Serious Disease like Heart and Stroke

Consequence Deficiency

*Increased Blood Pressure
*Increased Risk for Cardiovascular Disease

Iron Foods - recommended

*Beef
*Spinach
*Oysters
*Chicken
*Fortified Grain Cereals and Bread

Function

*Transports O2 through Body
*Memory Energy
*Deters PPD - Postpartum Depression

*Improves Bonding between Mother and Baby

Consequence Deficiency

*Birth Defects
*Extreme Tiredness
*Issues with Thinking and Concentration

Protein

If you want to be that super sexy stud muffin with washboard abs, or a toned and firm, lean sexy babe, sporting a slinky polka dot string bikini, they you're going to need lean protein **EVERY DAY!**

Protein is an essential macronutrient your body doesn't manufacture or store for the most part. It's vital necessary for optima growth and systematic function of your precious body as a whole.

Although the expert researchers and nutrition "wanna-

be's" of the world are still arguing over exact amounts.
The recommendation now is about 46 grams for women, add 10 grams for men.

If that number doesn't mean anything to you just think of it as 2-3 servings per day. Where a meat portion is about the size of a deck of cards, cheese is about an ounce, and beans would be a steamed cup.

Protein Foods

*Chicken (skinless - 17 grams/breast)
*Turkey (skinless - 17 grams/breast)
*Pork (23 grams/chop)
*Cheese (28 grams/ounce)

*Eggs (6 grams/egg)
*Nuts and Seeds (9 grams/ounce)
*Soy Beans (29 grams/cup)

Function

*Building Muscle
*Proper Growth and Body Function
*Memory

Consequence Deficiency

*Potential Muscle Atrophy
*Impaired Body Function
*Liver Strain and Issues
*Muscle Breakdown

Water

According to the *University of Rochester*, water is your lifeline! A newborn has up to 75% of their weight in water. Adults have up to 60%. Water is essential to running every single system within your body, from circulating your blood through your internal system, to delivering vital nutrients, including oxygen to each organ.

Water reflects how you think and feel. If you are dehydrated energy levels suck, nausea may creep up, and your brain may be frazzled in thought.

How Much?

The technical response considers:

*Age, Height, and Weight
*Activity Level
*Climate

*Basic Health
*Food Pattern
*Body Fat Percentage

I don't plan on getting technical, but in general experts agree 6-8 glasses of the clear stuff is the base of necessary **EVERY** day. You've got to use common sense, because if you're pregnant, or training like a maniac, this amount obviously needs to increase.

Your best bet is to start with 6 glasses and see how you feel. Carry a water bottle around to remind you to drink. You can even have a look at your pee, and if it's bright yellow you need more water. Unless you've just taken your multivitamin because that does wonders to the color.

Benefits...

*Transports vital nutrients throughout your body.
*Makes essential reactions in your body happen.
*Carries toxic waste from your body and kicks it to the curb.
*Aids in digestion
*Lubes up your joints
*Boosts energy

My Thoughts...

*Each of these essential nutrients are VIP for your body and mind to function optimally. By taking the time to en-sured you make a habit of eating healthy and get **ALL** of your essentials daily, you're going to provide your body with a solid platform from which to build a healthier you.*

*Smooth running and prevention is what it's all about...**YOUR CHOICE!***

Cathy's Important Point (CIP) - How you cook or pre-pare your food can seriously make or break a healthy dish. If you're adding butter and sour cream to your sweet potato you've created unhealthy. Eating a little salad with your dressing is disastrous. Frying, deep frying, creamy, cheesy, rich, sautéed in butter, drowned in oil, buttered, and mayonnaise, are all things to steer clear of when looking to get healthier with food.

Look to use condiments sparingly, where a tab of mustard, ketchup, barbecue sauce, or even honey mustard are acceptable. Look to poach, stream, bar-becue, bake, boil, grill, or broil your food. A piece of free-range chicken is healthy grilled, but deep fried or breaded is choosing nutrition-less calories and loads of FAT!

Chapter 5 - Consequences of Poor Eating - Benefits Healthy Munching

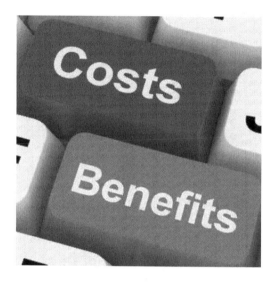

Unhealthy eating isn't something we really think about until we get slapped with preventable health issues. Sneaking a sweet treat every now and again, or going out for an unhealthy fast food meal once on a blue moon is **NOT** going to deem you an unhealthy eater with nasty consequences.

Unhealthy eating is something that manifests conse-quences over time, often years. Unfortunately it's poor nutrition habits that may jeopardize your life.

What you eat, how much, and when, affects every part of your being. How you look and feel, your energy levels, productivity, patience, life drive, temper, and will to accomplish.

Filling your day with dangerous Trans-fat loaded processed fast foods, pastries and cakes, sweets, donuts, cookies, candy, and other unhealthy saturated fat foods will interfere with your cognitive function, support weaker muscle and core strength, slower overall alertness, and so many other negative health consequences that interfere with a productive healthy life.

*Obesity
*High Blood Pressure
*Elevated Cholesterol
*Cardiovascular Disease
*Stroke
*Diabetes
*Various Cancers
*Mobility and Motility Issues
*Increased Chronic Pain
*Increased Illness in General

These are all directly linked with crappy eating over long periods of time. It's up to you to **CHOOSE** to start making healthier eating choices today so you **WILL** have a better tomorrow.

Benefits of Healthy Eating

*Increased Energy
*Decreased Risk of Disease
*Improved Mental Function
*Decreased Aches and Pains
*Better Chronic Pain Management
*Increased Optimism

*More Patience
*Less Moodiness
*Longer Life Expectancy
*Weight Control
*Stronger Heart
*Lower Blood Pressure
*Lower Cholesterol
*Faster Recovery Time
*Stronger Bones and Teeth
*More Efficient Internal Systems
*Better Brain Healthy
*Less Reactive
*Healthier Sleep

My Thoughts...

Understanding the consequences of choosing to eat un-healthy fat loaded convenience foods, and the benefits of filling your plate full of healthy lean means, energizing complex carbohydrates and minimal amounts of good fat, gives you the direction you need to create your plan of great sustainable health.

It's all about choice; turn left or right, or go straight through to healthier and happier!

Chapter 6 - Better Food Choices

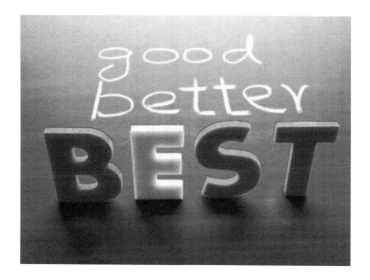

Do you prefer eating a white baguette or a slice of nutrient loaded healthy whole grain bread? Which is a smarter choice, a glass of juice or a bowl of fresh fruit? Would you pick a bowl of French onion soup, or a minestrone soup with a whole grain roll?

Every day you have choices to make on which foods you fill your cupboards and fridge with, what type of foods you snack on, and what ends up in front of you when dining out.

Here are a few "better" choices when making your food decisions!

Poor - White Bread   **Better** - Whole Grain Bread

Poor - Packaged Muffin   **Better** - 1/2 Whole Grain Bagel with Peanut Butter

Poor - Apple Juice   **Better** - Apple

Poor - Fruit Snack   **Better** - Piece Fruit

Poor - Salad with Dressing   **Better** - Salad with Dressing on Side to Drizzle

Poor – Pop-Tart   **Better** - Bowl Whole Grain Cereal with Milk

Poor - Fried Chicken   **Better** - Grilled Chicken

Poor - Mayo   **Better** - Mustard

Poor - Butter   **Better** - Olive Oil

Poor - French Fries   **Better** - Baked Sweet Potato

Poor - Energy Drink   **Better** - Water

Poor - Soda   **Better** - Water

Poor - 7 Grain/Multigrain   **Better** - 100% Whole Grain

Poor - Corn Chips   **Better** - Pretzels

Poor - Theater Popcorn   **Better** - Baked Potato Chips

Poor - Vitamin Water   **Better** - Water

Poor - 3+ Glasses Wine   **Better** - I Glass Wine with Dinner

Poor - Can of Ravioli   **Better** - Cup Pasta with Tomato Sauce

Poor - Pasta or White Rice   **Better** - Whole Grain Pasta or Brown Rice

Poor - Granola bar   **Better** - Handful Nuts

Poor - Chocolate Bar   **Better** - Chocolate Dip Granola Bar

Poor - Creamy Soup   **Better** - Clear Soup

Poor - Ordering Appetizers   **Better** - Skip Them

Poor - Bread Basket   **Better** - Send It Back

Poor - Nachos Deluxe chos with Salsa	**Better** - Multigrain Na-
Poor - Potato with Sour Cream or With Salsa	**Better** - Potato Naked
Poor - Egg Nog	**Better** - Chocolate Milk
Poor - Whipping Cream	**Better** - Cool Whip
Poor - Deep Dish Apple Pie	**Better** - Apple Crisp
Poor - Soda	**Better** - Diet Soda
Poor - Bacon	**Better** - Baked Ham
Poor - Double Burger	**Better** - Grilled Chicken
Poor - McDonald's Big Mac Hamburger	**Better** - McDonald's
Poor - Wendy's Angus Burger ior Chicken	**Better** - Wendy's Jun-
Poor - Poutine	**Better** - Fries
Poor - Macaroni/Potato Salad Coleslaw	**Better** - Non-Creamy
Poor - Bacon/Cheese on Burger tuce/Tomato on Burger	**Better** - Let-
Poor - White Bun Bun	**Better** - Whole Grain
Poor - Hot Dog	**Better** - Veggie Dog
Poor - Eggs Benedict	**Better** - Poached Eggs
Poor - Tuna in Oil	**Better** - Tuna in Water
Poor - Quick Oats	**Better** - Large Flakes
Poor - Frosted Flakes	**Better** - Shreddies
Poor - Breakfast Burrito with Ham on Whole Wheat	**Better** - Egg Whites
Poor - Assorted Sub Whole Grain	**Better** - Turkey Sub on
Poor - Bagel with Cream Cheese With Butter	**Better** - English muffin
Poor - Smoothie Fruit	**Better** - Yogurt with
Poor - Western Omelette Omelette with Ham/Veg	**Better** - Egg White
Poor - Oil	**Better** - Pam

Poor - Egg Rolls Soup | **Better** - Egg Drop

Poor - Fried Rice | **Better** - Steamed Rice

Poor - Sweet and Sour Sauce Sauce | **Better** - Hot Chilli

Poor - Deep Dish Pizza | **Better** - Thin Crust

Poor - Pepperoni or Sausage | **Better** - Chicken

Poor - Foot Long | **Better** - 6 Inch

Poor - Bacon Bits or Croutons Seeds and Raisins | **Better** - Sunflower

Poor - Extra Cheese | **Better** - No Cheese

Poor - Hard Taco | **Better** - Soft Taco

Poor - Refried Beans | **Better** - Black Beans

Poor - Teriyaki Wings | **Better** - BBQ Sandwich

My Thoughts...

It really is overwhelming knowing you can "always" make a better food choice. Even the healthiest health nuts in the universe can always improve their eating habits. The list above is meant to wet your appetite. To help set your brain up to make associations, helping you to figure out what's healthier even when you're not sure.

Just understanding creamy soups are faux pas will remind you to steer clear of creamy chicken or cream of broccoli when you can have beef barley or chicken noodle instead. Understanding you're better off having a whole grain roll than traditional soup crackers is going to move you one step closer to healthier eating.

Choosing lean beef over breaded chicken, or baked ham over fried pork, are little bits of food knowledge that will slowly but surely make gynormous positive changes in your waist size and overall health!

60

Commit to opening your noggin to change, making one adjustment at a time every day for the rest of your life. Promise yourself you're going to do that and results will happen FAST!

Chapter 7 - Action Plan that Starts with Food

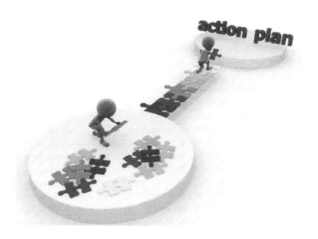

Creating a sustainable eating plan for life takes commitment and an acknowledgment new eating habits need to happen. It's important to understand your preferences and tolerances, know how much food your body actually needs, and learn to pay attention to your body signals.

Unlearning your poor eating habits and relearning fresh healthy ones is the wall you've got to climb, if you're serious about making simple eating changes in your life for fantabulous results.

ACTION STEPS:

Know Your BMI - You BMI is a calculation that gives you an idea of your body fat percentage. This enables you to see if you're in the healthy zone or not, and what course of action you need to take.

There are oodles of different BMI calculators online that take your height and weight, and determine whether your BMI is Underweight (below 18.5), Normal (18.5-24.9), or Obese (30+).

This method isn't 100% accurate but it will give you an idea of whether or not you're of healthy weight or not.

Know How Many Calories You Need - The easiest way to do this is look at a chart online. Essentially you'll need your gender, age, and activity level. From there the chart will give you the approximate number of calories you need each day to **MAINTAIN** your weight.

If your goal is to lose weight, with a combination of exercising more and eating less, you'll have to use up 500 extra calories for each pound of fat you plan on losing.

Keep It Simple - Counting calories and measuring food is tough. Keep ii simple by concentrating more of food groups and understanding portions as you move along. It won't take you long to recognize restaurants serve 3-4 times the portion you really need, so you can doggie bag it or portion it off early so you don't overdo it.

One Step At A Time - It's great to be all pumped to make all of your eating choices better. Set yourself up for success by understanding small steps that you can man-

age with your eating changes. That's better than gynormous ones that overwhelm.

If you're used to loads of butter on your white toast for
breakfast, try half that amount on whole grain toast until
you adjust. Then reduce it until you've just got a smear,
or perhaps are even happy with naked toast or with a dab
of peanut butter. *Health Today* says small manageable
changes work best!

Moderation Is Key – There's no one food decision that
will break you. But if you start overdoing it on a multitude
of poor food choices, this will steer you off track fast. If
you want some popcorn at the movies have a handful.
When cookies are your weakness, control yourself and
have just one or two on occasion, instead of the whole
freaking box!

THINK successfully - When eating it's best for your
mind, body, and energy levels, to eat 5-6 balanced mini-
meals each day. Make sure you've got lean protein,
complex carbs, and healthy fats in each one. This will
help keep your blood sugars level, deter mood swings,
keep energy levels up, and even deter junk craving because you're always running with your tank half-full,
instead of empty.

Visualize what you're going to eat on a plate if you have
to. Load most of your plate with healthy fruits and veggies, save a smaller portion for lean protein, and longer
term energy good carb foods. This will help you eat
healthy, provide your body with all the essential vitamins
and minerals it needs, and keep on track to lose weight if
that's your goal.

I wouldn't worry about getting enough fat. By eating a healthy diet in general and avoiding bad fat processed foods, you will give your body the healthy unsaturated fats it requires for optimal function without going over-board.

There's always the chance for too much of a good thing!

A small handful of mixed nuts is a great pre-workout snack. Making habit of having a whole jar is going to get you fat fast!

Make sure you never think in the terms of **FORBIDDEN FOODS**. Humans are competitive by nature and just don't like being told what they can't do. There is a little rebel in all of us!

If you can't pass up a piece of Black Forest cake that happens to come your way, understand you can have it if you really want it. The best way to do this is have two bites and flag the waiter to take it away, share it with someone, or commit to training an extra day that week to burn off the extra fat and calories.

You do have options.

The average small slice of Black Forest cake has about 400 calories. Which means an extra half hour going hard on the cross-trainer with ten minutes heavy weights, or a 45 minute spin bike class should do the trick.

Just don't beat yourself up over the odd treat here and there. It's the big picture that really counts.

Get Support - By literally shouting from a mountain top you are looking to make minor changes in your eating to lose weight, you're more likely to stick with the plan.

When life is throwing crap your way, having a friend or family member there to give you those words of encouragement you need to hear is priceless.

Plan Your Meals in Advance - For those of you who know me, I don't want to sound like a broken record but emotion and logic don't physiologically mix. If you don't have an idea of what healthy food you're going to eat next meal, and your tummy starts rumbling because you're delayed in eating, you forgot, or maybe just can't make up your mind, you're more likely to give into convenience foods.

Sweet cravings are triggered with hunger and your willpower isn't as resilient as when you don't have to consciously stress yourself deciphering between what you want and need to munch on. The physical needs of your body and the poor food choice habits in your mental will cause trouble.

By taking a few minutes once a week to forecast, or dare I say schedule your meals, you're taking action with simple measures to set yourself up for successful eating. We are lazy and don't want to have to think all the time, looking for an excuse to grab a candy bar instead of the fresh veggies and yogurt dip you packed in your man purse.

Think ahead, plan your eating, and you're ten pounds ahead of the skinny-wanna-be's that are confused and dazed trying to think about what they're going to eat while their stomachs are running on fumes.

No excuses here. Time for you to get *Martha Stewart*-like and begin planning, just stay away from trading!

Have Healthy Snacks Available – It's time to take action and make it easy for you to munch on the home-made trail mix you popped into your Holly Hobby lunch pail, instead of scootering over to the variety store on your shiny red Vista 6 volt scooter to grab a slushy and a bag of nacho chips.

Fill your fridge with whole food snacks, apples and oranges, fresh lean chicken, eggs, kale, carrots, milk, yogurt, and other grab n'go foods, so you're not trusting your free-thinking brain when you realize it's noon and you haven't had breakfast yet.

Shame on you!

Doesn't Sting to Consult Nutrition Expert - Particularly if you're straight off the candy truck instead of the turnip truck, it won't hurt to talk with a food specialist to help get you started. This could be a friend, your boy-toy who happens to be a nutritionist, a dietician, your doctor, a friend health nut, or perhaps a random stranger that looks to have more qualified food knowledge than you.

Any new piece of information you learn to make your food choices better makes it all worthwhile.

Keep a Food Diary - Don't even start whining to me with this one. The American Food and Nutrition Council unanimously agree keeping a food journal increases your success conversion rate.

It's a tool that gives your eyes satisfaction. Would you like me to describe the super-hot redhead dancing on the tables at Starbuck's in Collingwood, in her lacy black baby-doll, with spiked red heels, fishnet stockings, and a steel studded leather collar? Or would you rather just have a look for yourself before she gets hauled away to her new home?

Seeing is believing!

A food journal with keep you focused and paying closer attention to your food choices, simply because it hold you accountable.

Set Up Reward - Just like a puppy dog, you like a pat on the head, scratch behind the ears, or perhaps even a belly scratch now and again for good effort. Intermittent reward is a natural motivator to inspire you to choose the apple instead of a Twinkie, the whole grain sub instead or a deep fried squid rings, or a bowl of air popped naked popping corn, instead of theater popcorn with triple flooded Trans-fat poison.

Maybe after a week of positive health change, you're going to reward yourself with a new little black dress, or maybe even a night out with the girls to see the Chippendales live? If you need reward sooner, after each successful better eating decision that of course you noted in your gold satin good journal your boy-toy puts a buck in the pot to eventually buy you something sparkly for your efforts.

It really doesn't matter what the reward is. Just that it needs to suit your wants, needs, a deeply delicious desires. With the sole purpose of motivating you with a smile.

Visual Reminders Towards Measurable Goals - In order for most people to stay on track toward better eating, they need to create measurable goals. This could be weighing yourself once a week because your goal is to

69

drop 10 pounds by Christmas, which is just 6 weeks away.

Some people will check in with themselves by how their clothes fit. More loose is the goal, whereby snug means try harder.

You can also use your food journal. It shows you day by day exactly what you're eating, and seeing all that positive change is up-lifting.

Posting sticky notes on your fridge reminding you to eat your fresh fruit and yogurt for breakfast, is another fantabulous route to fire up your success rate with smarter food choices.

My Thoughts...

Oodles of people have great intentions to drink light beer, choose a grilled chicken salad instead of honey garlic chicken wings, or skip the dessert and go for extra steamed veggies, but never set out a plan to rake action and hold themselves accountable.

It's all about choice. Figure out your soft spots and poke them till it doesn't matter anymore. That's when you know you're serious about taking action steps with small changes and gynormous results.

Chapter 8 - Other Factors of Consideration

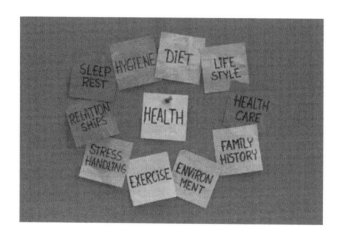

It's never ever in a zillion years possible to lose weight and keep it off till death do you part by just better eating choices. Sure that'll work up front for a few weeks, but trust me on this one, it doesn't take long for the honeymoon to end with that.

6 Main Factors Influencing Your Everyday Health Are:

Lifestyle - By lifestyle I'm referring to up close and personal activities and behaviors that influence your magical life.

Things like work, leisure activities, food choices, and social habits all fit here. Having a calm, safe, and somewhat stress-free work environment will positively impact your overall attitude towards better health.

Making sure you enjoy your leisure time regularly is a valuable part of good health. Going out bird watching with your nerdy neighbor is a great way to chill and de-stress. Striving towards making nutritious food choices will only fuel your desire and ability to get positive results.

Your lifestyle and positive life attitude are gynormously important in better health.

Exercise - I'm a biggie when it comes to regular exercise. This is something you just can't argue logically. Regular interval training physical exercise has been around since before caveman days. For cave-boys and girls it was a surreal part of survival. If they were fat blobs with slow reflexes, death was certain, particularly if a wild tiger invaded their cave in the middle of the night, moody and famished.

If these ancient day people weren't able to physically outmaneuver the dangers of their every day, or didn't have the muscle strength, motility, and coordination to hunt for food, carry water from the creek miles back to camp, make shelter, and walk hundreds of miles in search of fertile stomping grounds, they were literally **DEAD MEAT**.

Physical strength was the basis for survival. If you didn't have it you'd soon meet your demise. Even if you were in tip-top shape, if luck wasn't on your side, death was still a reality more often than not.

Times have changed and we live in a freaking techno obsessed lazy-butt society, where "convenience" should be our middle name. And I say all that with a big beautiful smile!

We get caught up in stress, make excuses not to exercise, eat oodles more food than we physically require for reasons other than innate hunger, and we make crap food picks for the sake of convenience.

THE RESULT? Fat lazy unhealthy eaters that look for excuses not to exercise, fast-forwarding the path to sickness, disease, unhappiness, and eventual death.

K - I'll stop there because I don't want to hammer society too much.

Exercise is something your body and mind requires for optimal health. At least an hour a day of intense interval weight training and challenging cardiovascular conditioning is where you need to start. Breaking crap-head habits is tough, but achievable if you make the choice to commit. Start small and work your way up. Experts say after 6 months of repeating a healthy new action you'll transform it into habit, which is exactly what the naturopath ordered when it comes to daily physical exercise with attitude.

Benefits of Exercise (According to the Ontario Ministry of Health and Long-Term Care)

*Lose Weight
*Sustain Weight Loss
*Deter Mental Disorders like Depression and Anxiety
*Levels Mood
*Boosts Optimism
*Triggers Patience

*Deters Disease
*Decreasing Annoying Aches and Pains
*Improves Intestinal Processes
*Supports Regularity
*Improves Sex
*Strengthens Heart and Lungs
*Increases Motility and Mobility
*Prevents Diabetes, Cardiovascular Disease, and Stroke
*Helps for Smooth Pregnancy and Delivery
*Builds Lean Muscle, Which Burns More Calories than Fat
*Tones and Strengthens the Body
*Improves Recovery Time from Injury
*Deters Injury
*Improves Cognitive Function
*Clearer Thinking
*Better Memory

Sleep - My friends at *WebMD* know all too well about the vital importance of getting quality sleep in relation to good health. Sleep deprivation will knock you down and take its toll on your physical and mental health over time.

Research shows lack of sleep is interrelated with just about every single health issue you can dream up. From colds and flu, diabetes and heart disease, to mental health and obesity, sleep is what you need to point your finger at.

FACT - Your body works 24/7 and needs to shut down at night for system repair and restoration. This means quality unbroken sleep for at least 8 hours EVERY night. To keep it simple, this can be broken down into sleep cycles, which happen about every 1.5 hours. This is just where your body goes through the 4 stages of sleep and is rested and restored when complete. However, if you are waking up at all hours of the night and breaking the process up, your body isn't getting the quality rest it requires, and you are going to be a cranky bugger to start, with sickness and disease eventually surfacing.

Most people do fine with 5-6 sleep cycles per night. And it's very important you set yourself up for great sleep habits, and figure out what's interfering with your sleep if this isn't your reality.

Question...Ever wonder why some mornings when your alarm goes off you pop right out of bed ready to go, and other times it feels like you've had no sleep at all?

Answer...Something as simple as waking up part-way through a full cycle, instead of when it's complete, can be the difference between night and day in how your feel come morning time.

Solution...**ROUTINE** is going to help you find your rhythm and for the most part make sure you get your health critical zzz's **EVERY** night.

Environment - Your environment plays a role in your overall health status. If you are living with a bunch of high-stress fighting maniacs or are always on heightened red alert, this is a toxic environment for you. When your workplace is loaded with toxic fumes and you're unable to get the clean air you need to breathe and function without feeling like throwing up your cookies, this is a crap environment for your health.

These are examples of environmental areas where you should look into bettering your environment. Not only for better health, but also a positive peace of mind.

Stress - Stress is a part of good health, but only to a degree. Our society reeks of stress and in extreme cases the health factor is all negative. It's not so important what the stressor is but how you handle it and perceive it.

Calm and relaxed, versus spazy and explosive, have two very different repercussions.

Stress ultimately dictates your path to disease, and often triggers unhealthy habits or coping mechanisms, like smoking, drinking, drugs, gambling, and even physical abuse.

Stress researcher *Bruce S. McKwen* of Rockefeller University states many things related to stress is a result of lifestyle choices.

Here are a few pointers to help manage stress and open the door to great health:

*Make decisions
*Write a list and cross of accomplishments
*Take time out for yourself
*Commit time for relationships
*Find time to go out with friends and laugh
*Make a point of helping others
*Commit to eating healthy
*Incorporate exercise into your life
*Take up new hobbies
*Enjoy your work or find something new
*Get the quality sleep your body needs each day
*Choose to be happy in life
*Surround yourself with positive

Chapter 9 - Final Thoughts

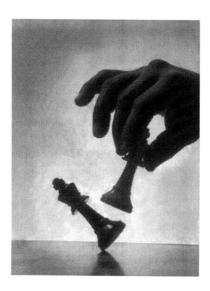

It all comes down to choice. If you don't want to or aren't ready to take action steps towards better eating and fantastico health, then you can't expect to look and feel better.

It Starts With Food is your first step in creating a resilient and continuously progressing life plan of better food choices and overall good health. By learning new healthy food choices, slowly but surely your old fatty processed fast food fuel source will soon become all but extinct in your world. It's up to you to take that first teeny tiny step toward change. Understanding that by continuing to make better food choices one by one creates a positive snowball effect.

You will experience gynormous realities that will quickly slap you in the face in the name of better health.

Fat will disappear, energy levels will shoot through the roof, aches and pains will diminish, disease will run away, your skin, hair and body tone will look amazing, your mind will focus positive, and you'll become addicted to making better food choices for life.

The seed of "more...more...more" will be planted and you'll look forward to doing anything and everything you can to get healthier and sustain what you've accomplished.

Adding regular exercise, stronger social relations, healthier environments, less stress, and better sleep and attitude to your big picture vision of smarter eating and fantabulous health makes results multiply.

One thing I can guarantee, is when you're ready to use this information and seriously make it happen, you've just taken the first steps to rest of your new and improved crazy-butt exciting and long-term healthy life!

Time to get to it!

Last Thoughts…

*THANK-YOU for reading my masterpiece. I hope you learned a little something, or at least got a few smiles.
*I would appreciate a millisecond or three of your time for a quick review, to help me build my masterful book empire higher.
*Whatever you do, don't forget to smile, and of course, check out my website for more of my e-Book masterpieces!
http://www.flawlesscreativewriting.com

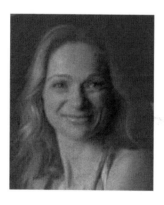

Cathy☺

Disclaimer

Made in the USA
San Bernardino, CA
30 August 2017